Sleep

I0408192

6 Techniques to Combat Insomnia and Sleep Like a Cat

by

Veronica Hurst

Table of Contents:

Introduction – page 2

The Dangers of Insomnia – page 11

The Benefits of Sleep – page 20

Sleeping Patterns – page 33

The 5 Stages of Sleep – page 39

Get Your Sleeping Cycle on Track – page 54

6 Foods That Help Stimulate Sleep – page 68

6 Techniques to Combat Insomnia – page 72

Introduction

Sleep is going to be an important indicator of your overall health and well-being. We actually spend up to one-third of our lives sleeping, and our overall state of "sleep health" remains an important question throughout our lifespan.

Most of us know that getting a good night of sleep is very important, but not enough of us make those eight or so hours in our bed a priority. For too many of us, we have forgotten the feeling of being truly rested.

To make matters worse, stimulants like energy drinks, coffee, alarm clocks, and even external lights including electronic devices block us from resting properly. They will interfere with our "circadian rhythm" or your natural sleep/wake cycle.

The amount you will need is going to vary with different ages and it's going to be especially impacted by health and lifestyle. To determine how much rest you need, it will be important to assess not only where you will fall on the "sleep needs spectrum", but also you need to examine what lifestyle factors are affecting the quantity and quality of sleep like stress and work schedules.

For you to get the sleep you need, you will need to look at the big picture.

The National Sleep Foundation has released their results of a world-class study that took them more than two years of research to complete. This updated our most-cited guidelines on how much you are really going to need at each age. You can read this research paper, it was published in Sleep Health.

Eighteen leading researchers and scientists came together to form the National Sleep Foundations expert panel that was tasked with updated the official recommendations.

The panelists included six specialists in sleeping and representatives from leading organizations such as Society for Research in Human Development, Gerontological Society of America, American Association of Anatomists, American Congress of Obstetricians and Gynecologists, Human Anatomy and Physiology Society, American Neurological Association, American Academy of Pediatrics, American Thoracic Society, American Physiological Society, American College of Chest Physicians, American

Psychiatric Association, and American Geriatrics Society.

The panelists participated in an extremely thorough scientific process that had included over 300 current scientific publications and voted on how much sleep is appropriate throughout our lifespan.

How much sleep is enough sleep?

Although research has not been able to pinpoint the exact amount of sleep needed at different ages, there's a universal understanding of acceptable time frames among experts. However, the determining factor is based on age rather than genetics or gender.

Nevertheless, it will be important for you to

pay attention to your own individual needs by assessing how you are feeling on different amounts of sleep. These are good questions to ask yourself to help you figure out a good amount of sleep for yourself.

- Are you happy, healthy and productive when you get seven hours of sleep? Or do you need nine hours of good sleep to get you into high gear?
- Are you overweight or at risk for any disease?
- Are you having sleeping problems?
- Are you dependent on caffeine to help you get through the day?
- Are you feeling sleep when you drive?

These are the questions you must ask yourself before you can find out the exact number that works for you.

Sleep Time Recommendations: What has changed?

The panel revised the sleep recommended ranges for all teen and children aged groups. These recommendations include:

- Newborns (0 to 3 months old): Their sleep range was narrowed to 14-17 hours every day (before it was between 12 to 18)
- Infants (40 to 11 months old): Their sleep range was widened two hours to 12-15 (before it was between 12 to 14)
- Toddlers (1-2 years old): Their sleep range was widened by one hour to 11-14 hours (before it was between 12 to 14)
- Preschoolers (3 to 5 years old): Their sleep range was widened by one hour to 10-13 hours (before it was between 11 to 13)

- School age children (6 to 13 years old): Their sleep range was widened by one hour to 9-11 hours (before it was between 10 to 11)
- Teenagers (14 to 17 years old): Their sleep was widened by one hour to 8-10 hours (before it was between 8.5 to 9.5)
- Young adults (18 to 25 years old): Their sleep range is around 7 to 9 hours (this is a new age category)
- Adults (20 to 64 years old): No changes were made to this sleep range it's still 7 to 9 hours
- Older Adults (65 and older): Their sleep range is between 7 to 8 hours (this is also a new category)

Improve your sleep today, make sleep a priority to yourself.

Most people don't realize the significance sleep has on your overall health. Your body needs time to rest, we are not indestructible. Sleep gives us energy to get through the day, and if we don't get enough sleep our whole days will be off. Do you ever have days when everything is going wrong and you can't do anything right? Did you get the proper amount of sleep on those days?

If you are wanting to start a new path towards healthier sleep and a healthier lifestyle, you will need to being by assessing your own individual needs and habits. Pay attention to how you respond to different amounts of sleep.

Notice how your health, mood and energy feel after a bad night's sleep compared to when you have a good one. Ask yourself if how often you are getting a good night's sleep. Just like exercise and a good diet, sleep is going to be a critical component to your overall health.

You could even try using the National Sleep Foundation Sleep Diary to help you keep track of your sleeping habits over a one or two-week period and if you have a physician you could bring the results to them.

But most importantly, you need to make sleep a priority. You must schedule time for sleep like any other daily activity. Do not make it a thing you only do after you get everything else done, stop doing other things over getting the sleep you need.

The Dangers of Insomnia

Sleep deprivation will cause damage to your body during short term. But over time it could lead to having chronic health problems and negatively impact your quality of life.

You actually need to sleep as much you would breathe and eat. While you are sleeping, your body is still working and tending to your mental and physical health and is getting you prepped for another day.

In children, and adolescents, while they are sleeping, hormones that promote growth are being released. These hormones will help in building muscle mass and they will also repair tissues and cells. Sleep is going to be vital for them so they can develop during puberty.

When you are being deprived of sleep, your brain cannot function right, which affects your emotional state and cognitive abilities. If this continues for long enough, it could lower your body's defenses, which will put you at risk for developing chronic illness.

The signs that are more obvious when someone is suffering from sleep deprivation are irritability and yawning. Long-lasting sleep deprivation could interfere with your decision-making abilities, balance, and coordination. You're putting yourself at risk to fall asleep during the day, even if you try your best to fight it. Stimulants such as caffeine are not capable to override your body's need for sleep.

When you are depriving yourself of sleep, the effects of alcohol are going to be magnified, as is the risk of being involved in an accident. There was a study done by Harvard Medical School that shown sleeping less than five hours a night will increase your risk of death from all causes by around 15 percent. Not getting enough sleep is dangerous to your physical and mental health and could dramatically lower your quality of life.

Central Nervous System and Lack of Sleep

Your central nervous system is what guides your body. Sleep is needed for it to function properly. While you sleep, your brain rests busy neurons and forms new pathways so you will be ready to take on the next morning. In young adults and children, their brains release growth hormones while they sleep. During your sleep cycle, your body is also producing proteins that are helping repair any cell damage.

When you deprive of the sleep it needs, it's going to feel exhausted, so it won't perform its duties as well. And of course, the most obvious effect is going to be sleepiness. You could find yourself feeling sluggish or yawning a lot. Not giving your body enough sleep is going to interfere with your ability to concentrate and learn new things.

It even has the ability to negatively impact both your long-term and short-term memory. It will get in the way of your decision-making and it will stifle your creativity. Your emotions will also be affected, this makes it more likely for you to have a short temper and mood swings.

If you deprive your body for long enough, you're will be in an increased risk of having hallucinations, especially if you have narcolepsy. Having lack of sleep will also trigger mania in people who suffer from manic depression. Other risks are going to include suicidal thoughts, impulsive behavior, paranoia and depression.

One of the side effects of sleep deprivation is micro sleep. That is when you are asleep for just a few seconds or a few minutes, but you don't realize it. Micro sleep is completely out of your control and could be extremely dangerous when driving or operating machinery. The National Heart, Lung, and Blood Institute has stated insufficient sleep has played a part in heartbreaking accidents that involved ships, airplanes, and even nuclear reactor meltdowns.

Immune System

While you are sleeping, your immune system will produce protective cytokines and infection-fighting cells and antibodies. These tools are used to fight off unknown substances like viruses and bacteria. The cytokines and other substances that are protective also help you sleep, which gives your immune system more energy so it can defend against illnesses.

When your body is not getting enough sleep

your immune system won't have the change to build up its forces. According to studies done by the Mayo Clinic, they have shown that if you don't get enough sleep, it's more likely that your body will not be able to fend off any invaders. It could cause you to take longer in recovering from illnesses. When you have long-term sleep deprivation it will raise your risk of developing chronic illnesses such as cardiovascular diseases and diabetes.

Respiratory System

Since sleep deprivation will weaken your immune system, you will also be more vulnerable to having respiratory problems like influenza and the common cold. If you have already been diagnosed with lung disease, sleep deprivation is likely to make it more serious.

Digestive System

Per a few studies that was done by Harvard Medical School, there was a link found between lack of sleep and gaining weight. Alongside with eating too much and not exercising, sleep deprivation is one of the risk factors to obesity.

When you don't give your body the sleep it needs that will increase the production of the stress hormone cortisol. Not sleeping enough will lower your levels of the hormone called leptin, which communicates to your brain when you've had enough to eat. It will also raise the levels of a biochemical called ghrelin, which is an appetite stimulate.

Sleep deprivation will promote your body to

release higher levels of insulin after you eat some food, this will promote fat storage and increases your risk of developing type 2 diabetes.

Cardiovascular System

Sleep is going to play an important role in your body's ability to repair and heal your heart and blood vessels. Not getting enough sleep could lead to higher risks of chronic health problems like stroke, high blood pressure, and heart disease. Per to a study that was done by Harvard Medical School, people with hypertension who have one night without enough sleep could cause elevated blood pressure all throughout the next day.

The Benefits of Sleep

For a long time, researchers were not exactly sure why we would sleep. There are several different theories that have been made over time. For instance, some are evolutionary, sleep will keep us out of trouble at night and keeps us away from animals who hunt after the sun goes down. But there are some that are physiological. Sleep helps us conserve precious energy.

There are some that are anecdotal. We need sleep to have a much-needed break to regenerate. In reality, our brain does a lot of work while we are sleeping, even though we are unconscious, our brain is still on. Just because we are asleep does not mean our brain stops working.

The RAND research group recently came out with a 100-page analysis on how sleep affects us and what sleep deprivation can do to use and our economy. They have estimated that between poor performance and lost work from lack of sleep, in the U.S alone costs us $411 billion every year.

Research that has been done lately has laid out some of the reasons why we are needing sleep, and all of our brain functions seem to perform while we are sleeping. There's a lot more to figure out, but here are some reasons why our brains need sleep, and why if we don't, things go downhill.

Sleep is going to help solidify your memory

One of the main functions of sleep is that it

helps you consolidate your long-term memory. It seems to do this, not only through strengthening our neural connections, but also through diminishing unwanted ones. The brain will make several different connections during the day, but not all of them are going to be worth saving. So, sleep gives our brains the opportunity to work through the information we learned through the day and decide what it really "needs".

Most people have most likely noticed how sleep will help us remember things that we have learned throughout the day. In one study, participants were asked to learn a motor routine by tapping buttons in a specific order. If participants in the study had the chance to go home and sleep before they performed the next task, they performed better in the same amount of time than the participants that recalled the tasks the same day.

This presents the theory that our brain stores memories it needs, and gets rid of the ones it doesn't. This is supported by research that has been conducted, it showed that the brain will tend to weaken the connections that form the memories that our brain see as unimportant.

One thing to be aware of though is, that sleep also seems to nail down negative memories, which could play a role in depression and PTSD. A recent study has showed that once negative emotional memories are integrated during sleep, they are less likely to be suppressed. So, this means that bad memories in addition to good ones will be more likely to stick around, and less likely to have been forgotten.

Toxins, even ones that are associated with Alzheimer's disease, are being warded off during we sleep.

One of the most fascinating discoveries over the last few years is that the brain clears out toxins faster while we are asleep than when we are awake.

The space between brain cells expands largely during sleep, which facilitates the clearing of the "gunk" in our brains, this is done through cerebrospinal fluid. Possibly one of the most astonishing facts is that most of this gunk is a β-amyloid protein, which is a forerunner to the plaques in Alzheimer's disease. Other toxins and proteins seems to gather up during the day, but they are cleared while we sleep. This is another incredibly reason to make sure that we get enough.

Sleep is necessary for cognition

It doesn't take a study to convince us that lack of sleep is going to affect our cognitive capacities, but luckily, there are several of them. Sleep deprivation could affect everything from attention to decision-making and cognition.

Sleep is needed for higher cortical function, and the most important which is multi-tasking, not getting enough sleep is going to affect that. Driving is one of the most intensive multitasking activity that we do, it uses our vision, hands, feet, and awareness of what's going on.

When you are deprived of sleep, it will strongly affect your ability to multitask. That is why we have so many accidents that involve cars, and of course, trains. Sleep deprivation will drain your executive function.

It has also been shown that sleep deprivation will have a negative impact on cognitive functions like working memory and attention. One study was able to find that just even a little sleep deprivation, the loss of 2 hours of sleep every night for 14 days, left participants with a weaker performance on certain neurobehavioral tasks that would involve short-term memory and attention.

If you want to be creative, your brain is going to need sleep

Sleep seems to spawn creativity, but sleep deprivation will strip it away. When people are being sleep-deprived, certain kinds of thoughts are going to be affected more than others. For example, divergent thinking, thinking in new and imaginative ways, thinking outside the box, seems to be the first thing that will go when someone is sleep deprived. But in convergent thinking, being able to figure out the right answer, like on standardized tests, will stay intact.

There was a study that deprived participants of sleep 32 hours and tested them on different aspects of thinking. People who didn't get sleep for 32 hours significantly did worse on most forms of divergent thinking, that included originality, fluency, and flexibility. They had the tendency to recall verbal memory tests. With this case, they were able to come up with the same answer again and again. This is a sign that the creative mind is actually not doing so well.

But on the flip side, sleep appears to be able to promote creativity. There was another study that had participants learning a task that involved numbers, in which they had to find a hidden pattern in the questions. People who got a good night of sleep were more successful at figuring it out than people who didn't have very much sleep.

Aside from all the studies, experiencing creative insights while you sleep, or just as you are waking up, has been documented for several hundred years.

Depression and sleep loss are intertwined

Depression has been known to be directly

linked to sleep deprivation. People who suffer from depression usually have a hard time sleeping, or they could also sleep too much. It also appears to be true that sleep deprivation, if not causes the depression, but it could certainty worsen it.

Studies have been able to find that people who sleep less than six hours a night or more than eight hours every night are more likely to be depressed than people who are sleeping in the middle. People who have insomnia are more likely to have anxiety and depression.

Something that could be part of the explanation of these connections might be from that fact that part of our brains that controls the circadian rhythm (this is your daily sleep-wake cycle, and all of our body functions that depend on it) is disrupted in people who are depressed. This could possibility partly explain how depression and sleep problems could be linked.

Physical health and longevity

Even though the mind needs more sleep more than our bodies, there are several physical diseases and disorders it can affect. A new study was presented at the Radiological Society of North America's yearly conference that found when health professionals had an average of three hours of sleep during a 24-hour shift, their hearts were suffering from it. The participant's contractility of their hearts had increased, blood pressure, levels or thyroid, heart rate and the stress hormone cortisol were all increased also.

There have been other studies that have been

able to link lack of sleep to obesity and overweight, and having poorer glucose control. Lots of studies have also been able to link poor sleep to mortality, but there seems to be a certain spot, if people get under six hours they are at greater risk, and those who are getting more than nine hour of sleep are night are at risk. The hormones mentioned above are likely to have to do with the effect of sleep deprivation, they can increase diabetes and heart risk, as well as inflammation, which could increase the risk of cancer.

Your sleep-wake cycle has an important impact on all our organ systems. We cannot deny the fact that sleep-wake pattern will affect the whole body, not just our brain. The most direct function of sleep does appear to be its effects on our central nervous system.

But we shouldn't ignore the fact that it does impact our body's organs.

Sleeping Patterns

Our sleeping patterns are hard wired based on a magical clock called the circadian clock. This pattern is known to operate on a "daily" level. It influences when you get tired and when your body wakes up. It controls how alert you are as well as the production of hormones, the temperatures of the body, how well organs are working, and even our sleep. This daily cycle is strongly manipulated by light, but can also be majorly affected by our body temperatures. When the body starts cooling off, it's easier for us to drift into sleep. If the temperature of your body is raising, you're going to be more alert.

A great example to back this up is to look at your body temperature before and after a meditation session and a work out. This simple test will allow you to come to grips with the managing of our temperatures. But temperature levels are only one aspect to this rhythm that helps control our major sleeping cycle.

The circadian rhythm is the biological clock that our body is genetically tuned, but our environment can also play a major role inside of energy levels and our ability to sleep throughout the day!

Every day, our circadian cycles control how much of energy that we have throughout the day, and can control our ability to become productive while simultaneously becoming responsible for making us tired.

Have you ever been tired, fought to stay up to a certain time, and then not be able to sleep? This is due to our biological rhythms that exist inside of our body. Today, we're flooded with technology, and we may forget the importance of paying attention to your biology and life so we can produce the sleeping results we so desperately want in our lives.

All of these sleeping prescriptions, software, and technology to help us sleep better is entirely useless if we can't master our own internal clock. Mastering your circadian sleep cycle takes work, patience, persistence and perseverance in order to overcome our challenges revolved around sleeping. However, it's definitely not impossible to achieve a great night's sleep!

The circadian rhythm is a major factor in sleep but we also have a major that rules our sleeping life called the sleep-wake process.

We have some rulers that help our biological rhythms. Cues from the environment that make major impacts on our body include the sun, aromas, and food consumption.

Another major factor that affects our overall rhythms are the schedules that run our life like school, work, entertainment, family interaction, and spending time with friends. As a result of all of the external factors that we can encounter inside of our daily life, it's easy to see how we could accidentally mess our body's sleeping cycle up with the time of day that it actually is. Overall, we have a massive system filled with checks and balances of our organs as well as the external feedback we encounter throughout the day.

This overall process has allowed us to create incredible feats throughout the evolution of man. The main manager of this process is called the suprachiasmatic nucleus.

It serves us as our master clock, and serves kind of like our overall operating system for life. It helps us "rest" when we have to and function at a certain level of performance when it's necessary throughout the week.

The suprachiasmatic nucleus, or SCN, runs through the communication of 20,000 neurons and is run by a series of receptors and "time cycles" that stimulate the activity of the body. Ganglion cells are the receptors inside of our eyes. While scientists are still trying to discover how the SCN system fully operates, our receptors directly communicate with the suprachiasmatic nucleus in order to help us manage our sleeping cycles. In other words, the moment that day breaks, our quality of sleep tends to decrease because our body becomes more aware of our external conditions.

The 5 Stages of Sleep

Traditionally, people encounter five major stages throughout our time asleep. They include stages one through four and REM Sleep. REM is short for Rapid Eye Movement. This is by far the most important area of your sleep. The stages of sleep are known to be progressive in order and go through from 1 to 4 before you dive into the dreaming stage that's responsible for regenerating your body, mind and energy levels. The standard for every sleeping cycle while we're asleep lasts about 90 minutes, but the exact number varies per person. Throughout every cycle of sleep, our brain shifts through different stages making for a dynamic performance from our bodies.

Even though these stages occur progressively

throughout the night, each major sleeping stage flux back and forth throughout the night.

Here's more of a break-down of each stage and how it affects your sleeping cycle.

Stage 1:

This stage is usually referred to as the stage that occurs as you're drifting in and out of sleep as you're tired. You can get woken up with relative ease while your body activity starts to slow down after a long day around the world! Throughout this stage, twitching is a common occurrence and it can even create a falling sensation inside of your body. This stage doesn't do very much for us. It's used kind of as a "portal" into our sleeping state.

Stage 2:

Stage two is where things start to get "moving" in terms of sleep production. Throughout this stage, our eye movements start to slow down even more and our brain frequencies start moving down. However, throughout the second stage, we can experience bursts of brain waves. These bursts of brain waves are known as sleeping spindles. They create a frequency between twelve and fourteen and are classified technically as sigma waves.

Another incredible phenomenon occurs at this stage called K-complexes. These complexes are interesting to say the least. They have short peaks of negative high voltage that's followed up with a more positive complex that finishes the K-complexes up again with another negative peak. Each complex lasts around one to two minutes.

As a result this stage of sleep, our sleeping cycle is protected. This is the stage where our circadian rhythm is less effective. Outside stimulus recognition becomes suppressed and is also responsible for help around the consolidation of our memories and experiences as well as the processing of important information that's been collected throughout the subconscious processing systems.

Stage 3:

Stage three is the result of the slowing of our sleeping during the preparation of your first two sleeping cycles. This important stage of sleep is commonly known as deep sleep or slow wave sleep. Throughout this entire stage, our environment becomes even less responsive. Thus, our awareness shifts from the environment directly into sleeping. This blocked out time occurs in longer periods of time throughout the first half of our sleeping cycle.

Stage three is known to be responsible for about fifteen to twenty percent of our total sleep time throughout our normal sleeping schedules.

We still encounter stage two sleep spindles, but they occur at a far lesser frequency. On the other hand, this stage occurs when our brains begin to produce delta waves that emit an incredibly low frequency compared to other first stages of sleep. Delta brain waves occur in frequencies of about half a Hertz all the way up to four hertz.

Stages three and four are highly connected because they both operate inside of the delta brain frequency. However, stage three is the point in time where our body is functioning at its lowest. Inside of this stage of sleep, your breathing becomes slowest along with the temperature of your brain.

This is also the time in the day that you encounter your lowest levels of heart rate and blood pressure. Stage three is the stage that's known as the most common state in which we enter our dreams without generating REM. These dreams are often vague and cloudy compared to our incredibly dynamic and vivid set of dreams that we encounter throughout our REM sleeping cycle.

Stage three is the stage of sleep that's

responsible for night terrors as well as sleep walking. If you've ever gotten little sleep and you've woken up groggy, this is typically the sleeping state that your body is encountering. The older you get; the less stage three activity occurs in your sleeping cycle. Toddlers tend to spend more time than adults, and seniors generate very little to no stage three sleep throughout the entire night.

Stage 4:

Stage four is typically the stage that the brain exclusively operates inside of lower data frequencies compared to the flux of increased frequency that can occur commonly throughout stage three. There's no body movement or eye activity compared to the other stages.

You can look at stage four like the calm before

the storm that's about ready to hit inside of the most important stage of sleep. Stage four has officially been classified as a variant of stage three, but these sleeping stages are known to be a little different in terms of stability in frequency.

Stage 5: REM

Stage five is where all the magic happens. This stage of sleep is dynamic, but it's also responsible for us feeling rested, awake, and alert in the morning. REM sleeping cycles typically blast out through ninety to one hundred and twenty minute cycles over the course of your sleep. In total, it's responsible for one fifth to a quarter of your sleeping time as an adult. Just like stage three, our REM sleep seems to decrease over time. Infants can spend up to 80% of their 14 to 17 hours of sleep inside of the REM sleeping state. That's a lot of dreaming!

REM sleep is the major driving force that occurs in the second half of our sleeping cycle. Every cycle we're asleep allows us to dive deeper into REM. If you've ever gotten cut short of sleep, it's because the hours before waking tend to be filled with REM.

Rapid Eye Movement is a stage of sleep that our mind runs absolutely wild. We encounter "random" and sporadic eye movements while our eyes are closed. To date, the only way to measure this stage of sleep is through the power of electrooculography, also known as EOG.

Our discoveries from this technology allowed experts to declare that our eye movements shift from tonic to a phasic state, but no one has discovered the reasons for this. It's my opinion that the rapid eye movement stimulates brain activity through the same communication channels that are responsible for the brain's interactions with stories. There is no concrete scientific evidence as to why we dream, but studying the brain's activity has given more insight to what happens with the brain while we are dreaming.

Dreaming and REM sleep may not be dependent. There are also alternative collections of research that indicate we may not even be "dreaming". What happens is that during the transition into our waking states, our mind encounters subliminal images that are being processed through our subconscious. In other words, our dreams can be the result of the language processing that occurs through subliminal avenues.

At this point in time, there is no other research that will aid in the understanding of this style of information processing. Eugen Tarnow indicated that this processing could be the compiling and processing of experiences into long-term support towards the overall experience that occurs throughout our major belief systems. Another bridge that supports this theory is the amount of time that children under the age of 5 are asleep. The increased time correlates with the research that indicated that our belief systems are mostly compiled throughout the first years of our life.

In other words, dreaming is the language of your subconscious using the power of story to create a dynamic processing of your overall belief system and its reactions to your experience. This same process is likely what's responsible for the regeneration of your body and every cell inside of it.

REM is characterized as a low-amplitude of different brain frequencies that reflect our overall brain processes while we're awake. It includes theta, alpha as well as beta waves that are used while we encounter focus and flow. This "paradoxical" style of sleep creates a condition where our brain encounters more energy and oxygen consumption than we do while we're facing a complex and challenging problems.

Our breathing encounters a similar situation as our eyes while we are inside of REM sleep. Our breathing shifts from slow and steady to rapid and sporadic as our heart rate and blood pressure rise with our brain activity.

However, there's one major factor that

separates our dreaming state from our waking state. Throughout REM, the physical body becomes entirely deactivated and our body becomes paralyzed. This situation is known as atonia, which is a result of your brain impulses that stimulate muscle movements are "disconnected" from your muscles. It's believed that the body is disconnected due to the powerful stimulations that fire off during REM sleep. It's thought to be a preventative measure to protect our bodies while our minds engage inside of "muscle moving" activities. Throughout sleep, if our brain doesn't receive enough REM, it is known to make up for the loss of REM at the quickest available time.

Throughout this stage of sleep, spatial memory consolidates as we acquire new skills. This is why people feel so tired after a long day learning something. While we're inside of these circumstances, we tend to encounter more REM sleep than we normally do.

Throughout our course of sleeping, we tend to wake up in very short spurts of a couple of seconds. We typically do not end up remembering these situations. However, if our wakefulness is triggered from the events, it typically takes an entire sleeping cycle in order to fall back asleep. This is why you find it hard to fall back asleep when you wake up through the night.

There's still a lot to learn about REM, however, we have a general feel on how the process works traditionally. This stage of sleep is crucial for us to function. At the end of the day, how much REM sleep we encounter directly effects how recharged we feel when we wake up in the morning.

Get Your Sleeping Cycle on Track

Developing a series of healthy sleeping habits can drastically impact your quality of life. Here's how to keep up with proper sleeping practices so that you can develop a good sleeping hygiene.

As you work on your transition into better sleep, you should expect to give your body and your brain time to adapt to the conditions. Sleeping patterns won't change overnight, and you should expect to get a little bit of lash back as your sleeping pattern and REM cycles shift with your new sleeping patterns.

Here are some wonderful ways to help you fix

your sleeping cycle!

1. Create a strict sleeping schedule throughout your week. Through following a consistent schedule you'll be able to live happier and healthier overall. If you consistently are changing what time you wake up and go to bed, you're drastically damaging your ability to develop a consistent routine throughout your life. This pattern can make you feel out of sync and off tilt. Having a consistent schedule will allow you to start taking control of your internal clock allowing you to bypass environmental triggers that would otherwise keep you wake.

It might feel great to have some fun if you've had a long work week, but messing with your sleep cycle may be the reason your work week was so hard in the first place. By giving your body the necessary amount of structured time it needs to generate enough REM to recharge your body daily.

Pick a hard bed time and wake up time throughout your week. If you love sleeping in or staying up late, you can use your weekends to ensure you have enough sleep. However, the moment your work week hits, it's crucial to run right back to your sleeping schedule. Staying strict around this method can be difficult. However, through using the other methods inside of this book, you can allow yourself to wind down before you drift off to sleep!

2. Use gradual adjustments. Changes are going to occur slowly. Unless you have a drastic shift in schedule occurring, it's best to scale back your bed time fifteen minutes every couple of days. This will give your sleeping cycle enough time to adjust to the fifteen minute periods. On the other hand, if you need to wake up at an exact time, but you're having trouble going to sleep, it's going to be important to develop a nice routine that allows your body to drift off to sleep more quickly.

3. If you have trouble setting up a morning routine but you want to, the best course of action would be to wake up with the morning light. Allowing natural light to drift into the morning will allow your circadian rhythm to spark up in the

morning. This will give you the perfect opportunity to make a hard set on your body cycle. This will give you the ability to fall asleep faster throughout the night as you adjust to your new waking time.

4. Always skip the snooze button. If you have to wake up at a certain time every day, there is absolutely no reason for the snooze button. Sometimes it can feel great to get that extra sleep, but this snooze ultimately ruins our chances of having a strict sleeping cycle that your subconscious can work with. Ignore the snooze button at all cost. Put your alarm across the room so you have to wake up in the morning. If that doesn't work, you can purchase a weighted alarm clock that only turns off if you stand on it for

whatever time that you want! This is a great way to wake up to one of your favorite songs and get a great start on the day.

5. Make sure your nightlights are dim. If you have a nightlight in your room, it may be causing you to get far less sleep. Our bodies were designed to sleep in the dark. By keeping a light on as you sleep, your body can have difficulties falling into immersive regenerative sleep.

6. While we're on the topic of light, the blue light that's emitted from our phones and televisions have the ability to keep us awake. In order to conquer this, it's best to turn off all of your technology one hour before bed. This will allow your mind to unwind and relax before you

start hitting your sleeping cycle. The more structured your time is, the more powerful your internal clock becomes. However it does take time to get there. There isn't much we can do about the aspect of time other than adjusting our sleeping times in fifteen minute intervals.

7. Pay attention to the times that you eat. Our body needs fuel in order to regenerate throughout our sleep, but being completely full isn't good for our digestive system. A consistent eating schedule around the evening will allow your body to tune itself to fall asleep when your food is digested. For snacks after dinner, a great snack would include carbs and protein blends. For example, cheese and crackers, protein(granola)

bars, and peanut butter banana toast are perfect options after dinner. As a rule of thumb, your last major meal should occur between two and three hours before bed.

8. Avoid substances throughout the evening. A nice glass of wine or a refreshing beer after work sounds great, but if you're looking to get your sleeping schedule on the right track, it's critical to stay away from substances after the late afternoon. Try to stay away from alcohol, energy drinks, coffee, caffeinated tea, and nicotine throughout the evening if you'd like to get your body in the proper state to induce sleep.

9. Develop a night time ritual to get to bed. A relaxing and calming routine inside of

dim lighting is the perfect way to clear your mind. Stress and thinking loops are insanely important factors toward our sleeping cycle.

If our minds are off racing or our body is filled with stress, it will have a heavy impact on how much REM sleep that we encounter throughout the evening. Stressors can cause you to fall asleep late or even stay awake during those small windows of consciousness after we awaken from REM.

By giving yourself a great window of opportunity throughout your evening to clear your mind, you'll be able to prime your body for sleep! A great evening routine would be to eliminate technology from your schedule an hour before bed.

You can start off with a brain dump through a journal. This will allow your mind to release the topic at hand and allow you to focus on relaxation.

After you're done with your journal, you can release yourself from all thoughts revolving around your life. Sit back and learn how to still your mind and embrace harmony inside of your body.

If you have trouble relaxing, you can follow your breath and make each breath slower and deeper. Focusing on your breath will still your mind, but you'll also cool down your blood pressure and your heart beat in order to create a better condition for sleep. The goal when we drift off into bed is to "deactivate" the stimulation of our brain activity.

10.   If you don't get good sleep throughout the night, don't nap. It may seem like a great idea to take a great nap throughout the afternoon, but the additional REM that you receive in the afternoon will cause you to need less throughout the night. This will put you in a situation where you get constantly put in a position where your quality of sleep will decrease during your night.

11.   Exercise on a daily basis. When it comes to sleep, working out every day is better than not working out at all. The more rigorous our exercise routines are, the better sleep they provide us as we hit bed time. However, if we finish our work outs anywhere under two hours before bed time, our body will not be in the

right condition for sleep.

12.   Manage the conditions inside of your room while you sleep. The temperature of your room should be between sixty and sixty-seven degrees. Eliminate all sources of light while you sleep so that you can sleep soundly, and ensure that your house is creating as little noise as possible. If you have a noisy house during your sleeping time, you can get ear plugs. If you have a room that is filled with light, you can get a sleeping mask! The less external stimulations that you receive, the better your sleep quality is going to be.

13.   Reflect on how good your mattress is. If your current sleeping situation is bad enough for you to study then buying a good mattress is of equal importance. The mattress market has developed incredible lengths since the last time you bought a mattress. If you keep everything else in your life the same, but you purchase a mattress that allows you to sleep comfortably, you'll undoubtedly encounter more restful sleep.

It isn't a scam when you hear people talking about how that new mattress changed their life. If your bed isn't keeping you comfy throughout the night, it's time you hit the mattress market. Make sure your pillow is comfy for you too! This may be a pricey road to travel, but a lot of mattresses have risk free trials you can take advantage of to make sure that you love what you get.

In other words, there's no risk for picking up a new mattress if purchase a mattress with a risk-free trial!

6 Foods That Help Stimulate Sleep

Food can affect our sleep just as much as it can keep us energized throughout the day. Eating the types of foods inside of this section will make you sleepy a little before you start your bed time routines!

Cherries

Cherries provide a good dose of melatonin, which is the hormone that helps control your sleeping and waking cycles. An extra shot of melatonin can put your brain into a good state to prepare for sleep!

Breads

Bread has a great source for carbs which creates a spike inside of your blood glucose levels. However, after you receive the burst of energy, you'll glucose levels will "crash" leading you to be sleepier. This is the same exact thing that happens to us after we have pasta for lunch!

Dark Chocolate

If you have a bit of a sweet tooth, you can take advantage of getting to sleep on time by eating a little bit before bed. People love to rave about the clean energy that you can get from dark chocolate. However, it contains a bit of serotonin inside of our brain that helps us relax. In other words it's the perfect dessert to top off your dinner!

Turkey

If you enjoy Thanksgiving, you might be in for a little bit of a treat. Meats like turkey have a good amount of tryptophan which is responsible for boosting your serotonin levels. Other meats you can dip into a little bit before bed are fish and chicken.

Bananas

Bananas are another wonderful way for you to unwind. The nice boost in potassium and magnesium help relax your muscles. This will also allow you to feel a little more sleepy and can help you drift off to bed!

Try Essential Oils

Essential oils are another wonderful way for you to dip into relaxation and serenity.

Lavender is known to be incredibly effective to relax your body and get to sleep. You can also use vetiver to hijack your body around bed time. You can apply these topically or aromatically inside of your bedroom! If you'd like you can even drop digestible night time oils into caffeine-free tea! Now that's relaxing!

6 Techniques to Combat Insomnia

Unless you learn to turn stress off, it's going to wreak havoc across your life. A part of the damages that occur from allowing stress to take over is sleeping. Everyone's been there. Life is stressful between work, family, and friendships.

It's impossible to rip stress out of our lives, but there is a point in time where we have to shut our minds off for the night. If we don't our mind can race a million miles an hour deep into the night. Stress can keep you up no matter what you do throughout the day. It's so impactful towards your sleep that there's an entire section dedicated to overcoming stress at night in order to sleep.

American Psychological Association declared that forty-three percent of adults stay awake at night due to stress. The same research went on to declare that almost half of the population is suffering from stress when it comes sleep quality by saying that the sleep is fair or poor. In other words, half of the population does not receive good sleep. Due to this circumstance, it's best to develop a nice routine in the evening that will disconnect you from your stresses. If you're not careful, stress can quickly develop into insomnia. It's believed by research placed in SLEEP journal that every single stressor we encounter increases the risk of insomnia by nineteen percent! This is because our body transitions from an active state into more of a calm state as we start to drift off to sleep.

When we encounter high patterns of stress, this system gets completely hijacked. It's understood that our sympathetic nervous system doesn't have the ability to shut down if we're stressed. Instead of getting the sleep that we need, our brain stays active.

This can lead to a massive onslaught of restless nights and can compound your stress even further. The only way to us to take control of this system is to ensure that we don't have any stress on our minds as we get ready for bed. Here's how to handle stress before bed so that it no longer destroys your quality of life.

Technique 1: Create a bedtime routine.

Create a routine inside of your evening for at least an hour before bed every evening. This will give you the time necessary for your body to adjust from light activity. Keep the room you're hanging out in as dim as possible (but still comfy) and turn off all the sounds and notifications on your technology. Watching Netflix to fall asleep won't work if it isn't doing the trick already. The most important part about letting go and creating a routine is taking control of your mind throughout the process. The first step to that is turning off all the chatter so you can focus on what matters most. The quality of your life!

Technique 2: Brain Dump.

Brain Dumping is a very popular and successful task in terms of productivity and is a prized asset among successful people.

However, the strategy is rarely brought up when we entertain our thoughts towards sleep. Having the ability to brain dump will put your mind at ease and will put you in the perfect way to unload all the stress you encountered throughout the day.

The idea behind brain dumping is simple. It lets you get all of those intense thoughts and experiences and allows you to put them down somewhere. Our conscious minds weren't meant to hold on to and entertain all the powerful experiences we encounter throughout the day. We now understand that there has to be a way for us to put our ideas somewhere, but where we actually place it is an important topic of discussion.

Some people genuinely document through technology. Others simply love sitting up a journal to brain dump. Personally, I enjoy freewriting for my brain dumps. I continuously write for the first 15 minutes of my evening routine to unload stress.

No matter what your preferred "style" of brain dumping is, there's a common system everyone can implement to create a successful brain dump.

1. Only use your actual handwriting.

    The first step in brain dumping is to actually dip out of the digital world and start using the power of language. Actively writing stimulates your subconscious mind in a fashion that is far superior to typing.

    Actually writing things down make them "stick" inside of our page and our subconscious. For some reason, it cements your thoughts and tends to allow you to release your conscious thoughts around a topic.

Take advantage of your current thoughts.

The first step in brain dumping is simply entertaining the thoughts that are on your mind. Fluently write about whatever's floating around and occupying your mind. This will allow your thoughts around the topic to expand and progress until you've "solved" whatever puzzle you needed to address through the power of fluent writing. Taking whatever you have and running with it is the perfect start for a brain dump! Just express all of the thoughts, ideas, projects, and stresses that you've let pile up inside your brain. If you don't brain dump on a regular basis, you'll typically encounter a style of "information overload". This will cause your mind to get intensified about subjects and can accidentally skip the triggers that shut our minds down for the day.

2. Know when to finish. The first couple of times you do this, you're going to be blasting out a lot of information. Sometimes, you're going to want to go on for hours blasting through all of your stress, thoughts, and ideas around life that you've been locked in throughout your consciousness.

   Knowing when to quit is a good point of time. Typically you'll know that your session is naturally done as you feel a pause inside of your writing "flow". To keep yourself in check you can set a timer with for the time that you feel like writing. It's recommended that you write for about half an hour unless you're dedicating over an hour. Brain dumping may be a great way to get all that locked up information inside of us, but it also stimulates your mind pretty heavily. If you find yourself writing past the half hour, you can choose to add more time to your evening ritual!

3. Focus on finishing ideas a little more quickly. Obviously we have dynamic emotions, but we can tend to linger around emotions and circumstances that can't currently address. By recognizing and expressing your emotion around a circumstance, you've let it blow off some steam.

There's probably something that you're hung up on. However, you're far less likely to discover this emotion today than you are in the future.

4. That's why it's important to come back to this writing routine daily. By consistently brain dumping, you'll be able to free up some space inside of your mind. Going through this routine 15 minutes a day has been more of an effect because it prioritizes the releasing of stress in between every rest rather than letting it pile up over a couple of days. Using this brain dumping isn't a fool proof solution. However, it's a wonderful way to release the thoughts that are stressing you out.

Technique 3: Remind yourself that you're not in danger and document your blessings.

After you brain dump, it's nice to still your mind for a moment before you tell yourself

"I'm not in any direct danger." This will allow to feel safe and present. You can do this for a moment and then count your blessings for about five minutes. This will put you in a wonderful mood after you brain dump. By controlling what situation you let your mind drift through, you'll be able to stimulate a circumstance that makes your feel more relaxed and comfortable. Having a nice state of mind where you feel safe, secure, comfortable and grateful is a wonderful state to be in.

Technique 4: Relax

Sit back and follow your breath for a while. You don't have to count if you don't want to, but it can help some people fall asleep. The act of simply following your breath until you drift to sleep is very effective once you have an established schedule.

However, if you're transitioning schedules you may find that you have a little trouble going to sleep. When this occurs it's very tempting to get up and move around. However, you should be in the perfect place mentally for sleep. The longer it takes for you to fall asleep following your breath, the more progress you'll be making in setting your sleeping schedule in stone!

Technique 5: Stay consistent.

Staying consistent with your evening routine is the only way that you're going to see results over time. Sleeping cycles don't change overnight.

Just because you started a new routine doesn't mean that your body has had time to adjust to it. If you want to make a lasting impact on your quality of sleep, you're going to have to be patient. Switching your sleeping cycle is known to be one of the hardest habitual changes that we encounter throughout life.

By sticking to your evening routine no matter what, your brain will react relatively quickly compared to you switching your schedule back and forth. Sometimes, you may find that you wake up earlier than you expected during your sleeping cycle. If it happens to be within an hour window of your desired schedule, you can simply wake up. This will help your mind set harder times your "inner" clock that revolve around your desired schedule. Drifting off back asleep for an hour can cause you to feel a little tired and groggy. By waking up when your brain is completed with the last cycle of sleep, you force it to work with the time that you have available. This will allow your sleeping cycle better adjust to the bed times that you're enforcing the next night! By doing this, you may be a little extra tired during the last part of the day, but that's a good thing if you want to get to bed on time!

Technique 6: Eat a recommended food

If you're still having a little bit of trouble, you can dip into one of the recommended foods half an hour before you begin your nightly routine.

This will give you that nice extra boost to put your brain and body into the right state as you drift off to sleep. Once again, any trouble that you're having falling asleep will automatically correct over time.

You realistically may struggle as you create

a healthier routine. When this happens, it feels frustrating. However, this is temporary. By committing yourself to getting to sleep at the same time every day, you're putting your quality of life first.

Getting great sleep throughout the week has some incredible benefits! By nature, the benefits of having high quality sleep are inverse of the negative side effects that are generated through sleep deprivation. This is due to the nature of the functions and restoration properties that occur from sleep.

This is just one example of an evening routine that helps you combat stress. However, it's important that your nightly rituals let you blow off steam, take control of your mind, and guide your brain towards sleep. Have fun installing these wonderful nightly routines into your life. By setting a hard time that you can stay up throughout the evening, you'll be able to always ensure you get wonderful sleep throughout the week. A well-rested life is priceless, but it does come at the cost of enforcing a solid and consistent sleeping schedule.

www.ingramcontent.com/pod-product-compliance
Lightning Source LLC
Chambersburg PA
CBHW062056280526
45788CB00003B/1249